CHROMOTHERAPY

- COLOURS AND WELL-BEING -

P.V.MIHALACHE

DEDICATION

This work is dedicated to my wife. You have made me stronger, better and more fulfilled than I could have ever imagined. Please do not ever doubt my dedication and love for you. I love you to the moon and back.

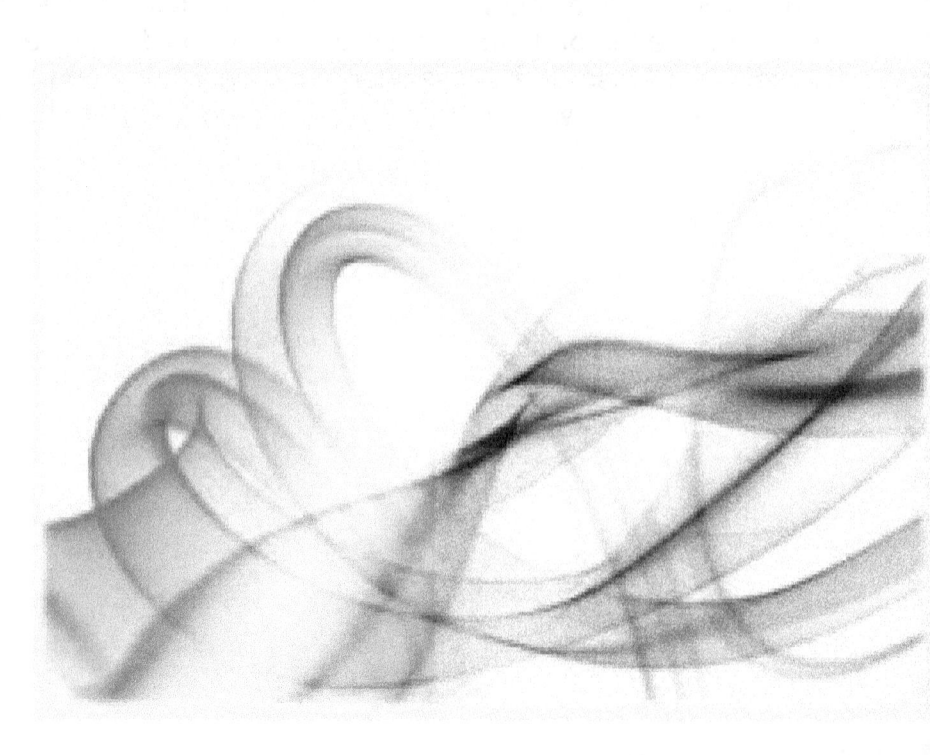

CONTENTS

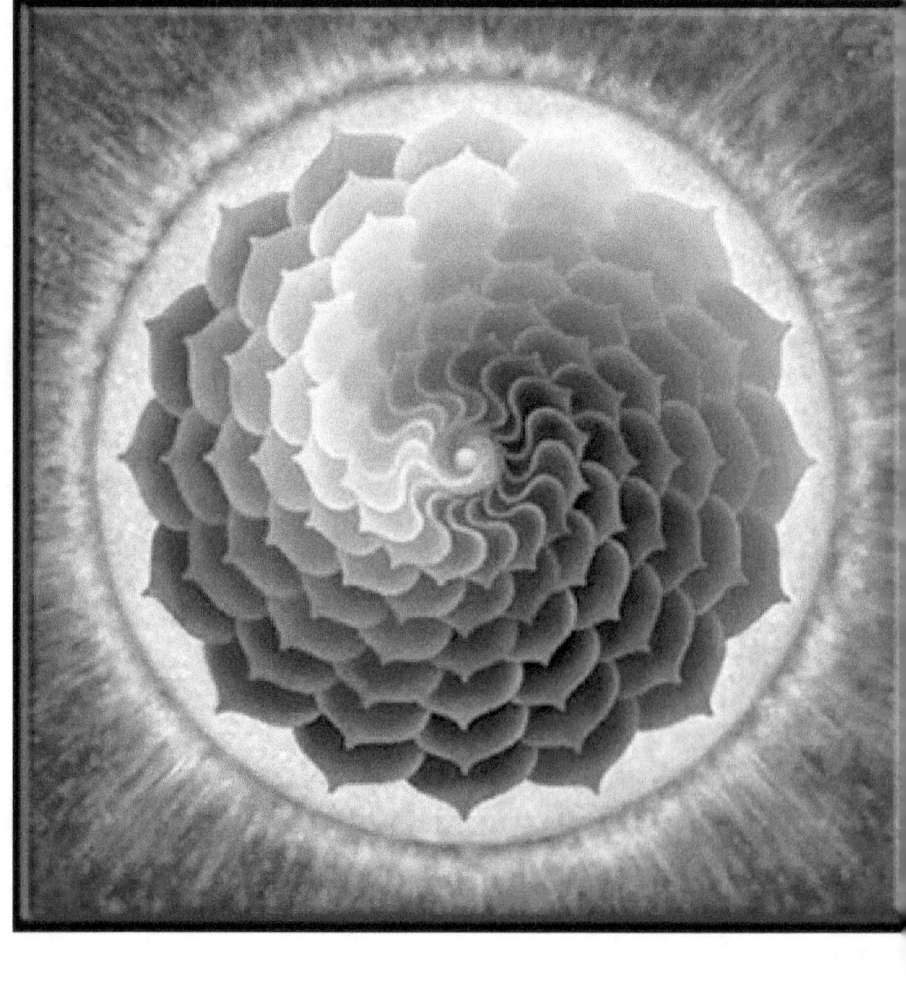

ACKNOWLEDGMENTS

There is evidence of people attempting to use colour for healing and therapy from as far back as 2000 years. And it has gained in popularity throughout the years, with numerous books being written about it, including JW Goethe who studied the physiological effects of colour.

As we mentioned though, many people are skeptical about using colour and light for healing or therapy.

1. WHAT IS CHROMOTHERAPY

Chromotherapy, sometimes called Colour therapy, Colourology or Chromotherapy, is an alternative medicine method, which is considered pseudoscience.

Colour therapy is distinct from other types of light therapy, such as neonatal jaundice treatment and blood irradiation therapy which is a scientifically accepted medical treatment for a number of conditions and from photobiology, the scientific study of the effects of light on living organisms.

Photobiology, the term for the contemporary scientific study of the effects of light on humans, has replaced the term Chromotherapy in an effort to separate it from its roots in Victorian mysticism and to strip it of its associations with symbolism and magic. Light therapy is a specific treatment approach using high intensity light to treat specific sleep, skin and mood disorders.

As most of you know, colour is light and energy. Colour is visible because it reflects, bends, and refracts through all kinds of particles, molecules and objects. There are a variety of wavelengths that light can be categorized, producing different types of light.

Visible wavelengths fall approximately in the 390 to 750 nanometre range and is known as the visible spectrum. Other wavelengths and frequencies are associated with non-visible light such as x-rays & ultraviolet rays. Most people are aware of the effects of non-visible light, so it makes sense that visible light would also affect us.

One example of the way light can affect us is a mild form of depression known as Seasonal Affective Disorder (SAD), which causes many people suffering during winters.

Colour Therapy is a complementary therapy for which there is evidence dating back thousands of years to the ancient cultures of Egypt, China and India. Colour is simply light of varying wavelengths, thus each colour has its own particular wavelength and energy.

P.V. Mihalache

The energy relating to each of the seven spectrum colours of red, orange, yellow, green, blue, indigo and violet, resonates with the energy of each of the seven main chakras/energy centres of the body.

If you can imagine the chakras as a set of cogs/wheels, they are rather like the workings of a clock or an engine.

Each cog/wheel needs to move smoothly for the clock/engine to work properly. Thus good health and wellbeing is achieved by a balance of all these energies.

Balance of the energy in each of the body's chakras is very important for health and wellbeing. Colour therapy can help to re-balance and/or stimulate these energies by applying the appropriate colour to the body and therefore re-balance our chakras. Red relates to the base chakra, orange the sacral chakra, yellow the solar plexus chakra, green the heart chakra, blue the throat chakra, indigo the brow chakra and violet relates to the crown chakra.

Colour	Chakra	Chakra location	Alleged function
Red	First	Base of the spine	Grounding and Survival
Orange	Second	Lower abdomen, genitals	Emotions, sexuality
Yellow	Third	Solar plexus	Power, ego
Green	Fourth	Heart	Love, sense of responsibility
Blue	Fifth	Throat	Physical and spiritual communication
Indigo	Sixth	Just above the center of the brow, middle of forehead	Forgiveness, compassion, understanding
Violet	Seventh	Crown of the head	Connection with universal energies, transmission of ideas and information

Colour is absorbed by the eyes, skin, skull our 'magnetic energy field' or aura and the energy of colour affects us on all levels, that is to say, physical, spiritual and emotional. Every cell in the body needs light energy - thus colour energy has widespread effects on the whole body. There are many different ways of giving colour, including; Solarized Water, Light boxes/lamps with colour filters, colour silks and hands on healing using colour.

Colour therapy and healing is a type of holistic healing that uses the visible spectrum of light and colour to affect a person's mood and physical or mental health. Each colour falls into a specific frequency and vibration, which many believe contribute to specific properties that can be used to affect the energy and frequencies within our bodies.

While it is common knowledge that light enters through our eyes, it's important to note that light can also enter through our skin. Given the unique frequencies and vibrations of various colours, people believe that certain colours entering the body can activate hormones causing chemical reactions within the body, then influencing emotion and enabling the body to heal.

Colours are known to have an effect on people with brain disorders or people with emotional troubles. The colour blue can have a calming effect which can then result in lower blood pressure, whereas the colour red might have the opposite effect. Green is another colour that may be used to relax people who are emotionally unbalanced. Yellow, on the other hand, may be used to help invigorate people who might be suffering from depression.

Alternative therapies also believe that a person's aura contains different layers of light which can be used for cleansing and balancing.

Knowing the colours in your aura can help you better understand your spirit, and thus help you better understand how to heal. Additionally, the colours surrounding you can also have various effects.

P.V. Mihalache

Colour therapy can be shown to help on a physical level, which is perhaps easier to quantify, however there are deeper issues around the colours on the psychological and spiritual levels.

Our wellbeing is not, of course, purely a physical issue. Fortunately, many more practitioners, both orthodox and complementary are now treating patients in an holistic manner. That is to say, we are body, mind and spirit and none of these areas function entirely alone; each has an effect upon the other. This is why Colour Therapy can be so helpful since colour addresses all levels of our being.

As babies we first experience colour in the womb where we are enveloped in a nurturing and comforting pink. Then as a child we associate with colour as part of our first learning processes. These first associations contribute to our consciousness. As we get older we attach many different feelings, memories and meanings to certain colours and this can then become a feature in our subconscious. We can build up prejudices to colours which have happy, sad, or frightening connotations for us.

All life experiences make an impression upon us. Some experiences will be positive and some negative. It is these negative experiences which can manifest themselves physically over time as dis-ease. As an example: perhaps we have, over the years, been in a situation where we have felt unable, for one reason or another, to speak our mind, or to express our own truth. This can manifest as a problem in the throat chakra. The throat chakra relates in the spiritual aspect to self expression. Thus, if our self expression has been blocked, the energy in this area will not be free flowing and in turn this can lead to a physical manifestation of dis-ease.

Noting strong colour preferences can also be a helpful aid to finding possible problems and working with the appropriate colour/colours to help to dispel negative feelings, free blocks and re-balance the body emotionally, spiritually and, in turn, physically.

Colour Therapy is a totally holistic and non-invasive therapy and, really, colour should be a part of our everyday life, not just something we experience for an hour or two with a therapist. Colour is all around us everywhere. This wonderful planet does not contain all the beautiful colours of the rainbow for no reason. Nothing on this earth is here just by chance; everything in nature is here for a purpose. Colour is no exception. All we need to do is to heighten our awareness of the energy of colour and how it can transform our lives. A professional therapist will help you to do this. The capacity for health and wellbeing is within us all.

Colour therapy is safe to use alone or alongside any other therapy whether orthodox medicine or another complementary therapy and is safe and helpful for adults, children and animals too.

Please be aware that no complementary therapy should be considered as an alternative to professional medical advice where necessary and no properly qualified complementary therapist would suggest that, neither would they suggest that you stop taking your medication etc. If you are taking medication you should consult the prescribing professional before you stop taking it.

Each of the spectrum colours is simply light of varying wavelengths, thus each colour has its own particular energy. The energy relating to each of these spectrum colours resonates with the energy of each of the seven main chakras of the body.

If you can imagine the chakras/energy centres as a set of cogs/wheels, they are rather like the workings of a clock or an engine; each cog /wheel needs to move smoothly and at a similar speed for the clock/engine to work properly. Thus good health and well-being is achieved by a balance of all these energies.

Colour therapy can help to re-balance these 'wheels' by applying the appropriate colour to the body and therefore re-balance our chakras. Listed below is each of the spectrum colours and the chakra which it relates to.

5

Colour therapy is classified as a vibrational healing modality. Vibrational medicine incorporates the use of chi energies within living organisms such as plants, gemstones and crystals, water, sunlight, and sound.

Colour is simply a form of visible light, of electromagnetic energy. All the primary colours reflected in the rainbow carry their own unique healing properties. The sun alone is a wonderful healer! Just imagine what life would be like without sunshine. It has been proven that lack of sunlight contributes to depression for some people.

A therapist trained in colour therapy applies light and colour in the form of tools, visualization, or verbal suggestion to balance energy in the areas of our bodies that are lacking vibrance, be it physical, emotional, spiritual, or mental.

We delight in a rainbow, sigh at a sunset, luxuriate in the rich colours of our homes, clothes, special spaces. Our eyes gravitate towards saturated colour like moths to the light. No coincidence, considering the entire spectrum of colours is derived from light.

And no surprise, really, that seeing, wearing or being exposed to colour- whether in the form of light, pigment, or cloth- can affect us at levels we are only just beginning to understand.

Scientifically, it makes sense. Colour is simply a form of visible light, of electromagnetic energy. Let's break it down. What exactly is light? It is the visible reflection off the particles in the atmosphere.

Violet has the shortest wavelength and red the longest wavelength.

Colour makes up a band of these light wave frequencies from red at 1/33,000th's of an inch wavelength to violet at 1/67,000 of an inch wavelength. Below red lie infrared and radio waves and above it the invisible ultraviolet, x-rays, and gamma rays. We all understand the impact of ultraviolet and x-rays, do we not? We all know the medical effect of this rays so why then wouldn't the light we can see "as colour" not have as big an impact?

Do you feel anxious in a yellow room? Does the colour blue make you feel calm and relaxed? Artists and interior designers have long understood how colour can dramatically affect moods, feelings, and emotions. It is a powerful communication tool and can be used to signal action, influence mood, and cause physiological reactions.
Certain colours have been associated with increased blood pressure, increased metabolism, and eyestrain.

How we "feel" about colour is more than psychological. The last decade has proven that lack of colour, or more specifically, light, causes millions to suffer each winter from a mild depression known as Seasonal Affective Disorder (SAD). Because of the complex way in which exposure to various colours acts via the brain upon the autonomic nervous system, exposure to a specific colour can even alter physiological measurements such as blood pressure, electrical skin resistance and glandular functions in your body. And they most certainly can affect how you feel on a day-to-day basis. Learning about colour's qualities and putting it to use can enhance your spirit, improve your health, and quite ultimately, expand your consciousness.
Colour therapy is used by alternative health practitioners who use colour to balance energy wherever our bodies are lacking, be it physical, emotional, spiritual, or mental. Angie Arkin, Intuitive Healer in Key West, uses colour during her sessions with clients, and often works with colour during her own personal meditations.

"Your aura is just an energy field that surrounds you," says Arkin. "In your aura, there are different layers, and in each layer, there are different colours that may be used for clearing and rebalancing your energy field. An aura reading is looking at the colours found in your aura. Knowing what colours are in your aura brings you closer to your spirit. If you can consciously bring that out, you have more advantage in clearing and healing your life. It's really just another layer of knowing."

Jasmine Sky, also a Florida Keys resident, brings healing and colour therapy to clothing. "Painting on silk and installing healing prayers into the silk seemed to marry all parts of me - the part of me that was a healer, the part of me that was an artist, my love of fabrics and many years of sewing, my love of tropical islands with sarongs being their indigenous clothing," she says.

Jasmine, having studied colour therapy, takes this into consideration when working with clients for their custom design. "Specifically I work with customers on the emotional space they want to be in, and recommend colours accordingly. This informs the prayers and Reiki symbols I paint in to the silk. And the silk itself has unique energy and healing properties. I also draw on my own intuitive resources to make recommendations." All this is part of the reason Sky talks to each customer before creating a garment, even if it is one of the standard designs.

Sky also refers customers to, and works with Arkin, in applying colour readings to garment design. They are currently working together to integrate Arkin's readings into The Dreaming Goddess Web site.

While perceptions of colour are somewhat subjective, there are some colour effects that have universal meaning. Colours in the red area of the colour spectrum are known as warm colours and include red, orange and yellow. These warm colours evoke emotions ranging from feelings of warmth and comfort to feelings of anger and hostility.

Colours on the blue side of the spectrum are known as cool colours and include blue, purple and green. These colours are often described as calm, but can also call to mind feelings of sadness or indifference.

Several ancient cultures, including the Egyptians and Chinese, practiced Chromotherapy, or the use of colours to heal. In this treatment Red was used to stimulate the body and mind and to increase circulation, Yellow was thought to stimulate the nerves and purify the body.

Orange was used to heal the lungs and to increase energy levels. Blue was believed to soothe illnesses and treat pain. Indigo shades were thought to alleviate skin problems.

Most psychologists view colour therapy with skepticism and point out that the supposed effects of colour are often grossly exaggerated. Colours also have different meanings in different cultures. Research has demonstrated in many cases that the mood-altering effects of colour may only be temporary. A blue room may initially cause feelings of calm, but the effect dissipates after a short period of time.

However, the existing research has found that colour can impact people in a variety of surprising ways:

One study found that warm-coloured placebo pills were reported as more effective than cool-coloured placebo pills.

Anecdotal evidence has suggested that installing blue-coloured streetlights can lead to a reduction of crime in those areas.

The temperature of the environment might play a role in colour preference. People who are warm tend to list cool colours as their favorites, while people who are cold prefer warmer colours.

More recently, researchers discovered that the colour red causes people to react with greater speed and force, something that might prove useful during athletic activities.

One study that looked at historical data found that sports teams dressed in mostly black uniforms are more likely to receive penalties and that students were more likely to associate negative qualities with a player wearing a black uniform.

Studies have also shown that certain colours can have an impact on performance. No one likes to see a graded test covered in red ink, but one study found that seeing the colour red before taking an exam actually hurt test performance. While the colour red is often described as threatening, arousing or exciting, many previous studies on the impact of the colour red have been largely inconclusive.

The study found, however, that exposing students to the colour red prior to an exam has been shown to have a negative impact on test performance.

In the first of the six experiments described in the study, 71 U.S. colleges students were presented with a participant number coloured either red, green or black prior to taking a five-minute test. The results revealed that students who were presented with the red number before taking the test scored more than twenty percent lower than those presented with the green and black numbers.

Interest in the subject of colour psychology is growing, but there remain a number of unanswered questions. How do colour associations develop? How powerful is the influence of these associations on real-world behavior? Can colour be used to increase worker productivity or workplace safety? What colours have an impact on consumer behavior? Do certain personality types prefer certain colours? As researchers continue to explore such questions, we may soon learn more about the impact that colour has on human psychology.

Zena O'Connor, a faculty member in the Department of Architecture, Design, and Planning at the University of Sydney, suggests that people should be wary of many of the claims they see about the psychology of colour. "Many of these claims lack substantiation in terms of empirical support, exhibit fundamental flaws and may include factoids presented as facts," O'Connor explains. "In addition, such claims often refer to outdated research without referring to current research findings."

So what's the bottom line? Experts have found that while colour can have an influence on how we feel and act, these effects are subject to personal, cultural, and situational factors. More scientific research is needed to gain a better understanding of colour psychology.

The Earth, our continents, oceans, in fact every living thing depends on light to be able to exist. Recent scientific evidence suggests that light is in fact emitted by every cell in our bodies.

We live in a sea of energy where colour is working within us. It shines with in our divine self, and radiates upon us from the sun. Research and observation has shown us that specific colours bring balance to our physical and emotional systems.

Chromotherapy can easily be used as an alternative to Chinese acupuncture, achieving the same results in unblocking meridians without the discomfort of needles used in acupuncture.

Carl Jung, a renowned psychiatrist and proponent of art therapy, encouraged his patients to use colour because he felt this would help them express some of the deeper parts of their psyche. It is believed that the colour choices you make reflect a deeper meaning about your personality traits. For example, introverts and extroverts are likely to choose different colours – blue and red respectively.

The colours you choose to wear might also say something about how you are feeling that day. Some days you may feel like wearing something lighter, something red, or something blue. These choices are often a reflection of how you are feeling at the moment. Additionally, wearing certain colours may cause you to react differently to certain situations.

There are two main sources of light that create the colours we see: the sun and lightbulbs.

As you know, the light from the sun allows us to see things during the day as well as during the night when the sun's light reflects off the moon. There is a visible spectrum of colours that we can see in addition to the combination of all colours (white) and the absence of colour (black).

Surfaces reflect and absorb light differently, which results in the colours we see through our eyes. For example, a tomato absorbs all light on the spectrum except the red rays of light.

The red rays of light are reflected off the surface of the tomato which then reaches our eyes for processing.

The coloured light enters the eye through the pupil, goes through the lens, and then reaches the back of the eye called the retina. On the retina there are a bunch of light sensors called rods and cones. These rods and cones send a signal to the brain about what the eye is seeing.

The cones are capable of seeing three colours: red, green, and blue. These are known as primary colours (RGB Model)

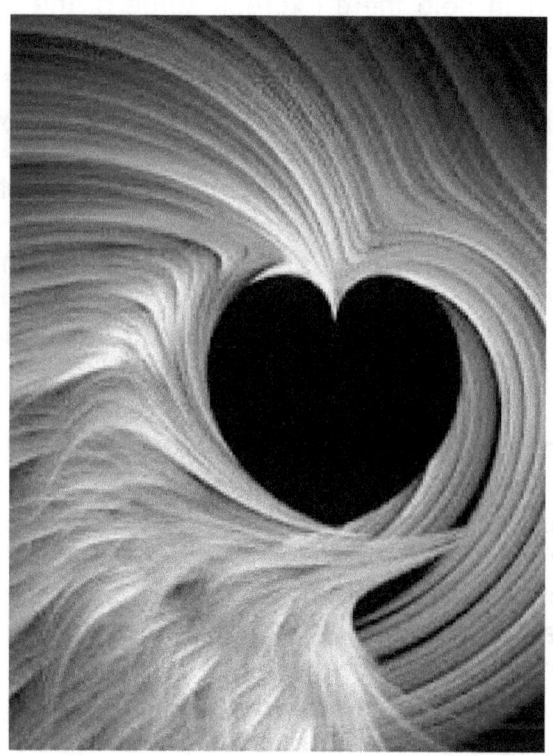

2. CHROMOTHERAPY HISTORY

This is no new news. Egyptians built healing temples of light four thousand years ago, bathing patients in specific colours of light to produce different effects. Now, before you begin to pooh-pooh the pyramids, consider these factual goodies. Research shows that a blindfolded person will experience physiological reactions under different coloured rays. In other words, the skin sees in Technicolour. Noted neuropsychologist Kurt Goldstein confirmed this information in his modern classic The Organism, where he notes that stimulation of the skin by different colours creates different effects.

Ancient observation Chromotherapy is a centuries-old concept. The history of colour medicine is as old as that of any other medicine. Phototherapy was practiced in ancient Egypt, Greece, China and India. The Egyptians utilized sunlight as well as colour for healing. Colour has been investigated as medicine since 2000 BC . People of that era were certainly unaware of the scientific facts of colours as medicine, but they certainly had faith in healing with colours.

They used primary colours for healing as they were unaware of the mixing up of two colours. The science seems to have been silent at those times.

According to ancient Egyptian mythology, the art of Chromotherapy was discovered by the god Thoth. In the hermetic traditions, the ancient Egyptians and Greeks used coloured minerals, stones, crystals, salves and dyes as remedies and painted treatment sanctuaries in various shades of colours. The ancient Ayurvedic physician Charaka, who lived in the sixth century BC, recommended sunlight to treat a variety of diseases.

In ancient Greece the physical nature of colour was dominant. Colour was intrinsic to healing, which involved restoring balance. Garments, oils, plasters, ointments and salves were used to treat disease.

The Greeks were unaware of biological changes in the body as a result of colour treatment; nevertheless, they had blind faith in the healing properties of colours. It is also interesting to know that they used both forms of treatment with colours: direct exposure to sunlight and indirect healing. In the indirect method, they used such materials as stones, dyes, ointments and plasters as the medium. What was missing in their medicinal use of colour was water as a medium for the absorption of colour, which later proved to be the best remedy for removing toxins from the body. This concept is common among all researchers working on hydrochromopathy.

Avicenna (AD 980) advanced the art of healing using colours. He made clear the vital importance of colour in both diagnosis and treatment. According to Avicenna, 'Colour is an observable symptom of disease.' He also developed a chart that related colour to temperature and physical condition of the body. He used colour treatment with the view that red moved the blood, blue or white cooled it and yellow reduced muscular pain and inflammation.

Avicenna's work undoubtedly advanced the use of Chromotherapy in those times. He discussed the properties of colours for healing and was the first to establish that the wrong colour suggested for therapy would certainly elicit no response in specific diseases. For example, he observed that a person with a nosebleed should not gaze at things of a brilliant red colour and should not be exposed to red light because this would stimulate the sanguineous humor, whereas blue would soothe it and reduce blood flow. This seems to be the practical understanding at the time, but we do not find discrete values of frequencies or energies associated with these colours.

In 1666, English scientist Sir Isaac Newton discovered that when pure white light passes through a prism, it separates into all of the visible colours. Newton also found that each colour is made up of a single wavelength and cannot be separated any further into other colours.

Further experiments demonstrated that light could be combined to form other colours, red light mixed with yellow light creates an orange colour. Some colours, such as yellow and purple, cancel each other out when mixed and result in a white light.

If you have ever painted, then you have probably noticed how certain colours can be mixed to create other colours..

American Civil War General Augustus Pleasonton (1801-1894) conducted his own experiments and in 1876 published his book The Influence Of The Blue Ray Of The Sunlight And Of The Blue Colour Of The Sky about how the Colour blue can improve the growth of crops and livestock and can help heal diseases in humans.

He used only blue and stated that blue was the first remedy in case of injuries, burns or aches. He reported his findings on the effects of colour in plants, animals and humans. He claimed that 'the quality yield and the size of grapes could significantly increase if they were grown in a greenhouse made with alternating blue and transparent panes of glass. He also cured certain diseases and increased fertility as well as the rate of physical maturation in animals by exposing them to blue light. The same methodology employing the colour blue was adopted by Hassan (1999), who found it to be very useful as a first-line treatment for injuries as well as for burns. Since, Pleasanton's work lacked scientific proof and evidence, no established rules were presented before the scientific societies, leading to a great gap between his work and the development of colour/vibrational healing on scientific grounds. If work could be carried out even now on his great ideas, especially in agricultural development and in animals, researchers could make new discoveries.

This led to modern Chromotherapy, influencing scientist Dr. Seth Pancoast (1823-1889) and Edwin Dwight Babbitt to conduct experiments and to publish, respectively, Blue and Red Light; or, Light and Its Rays as Medicine (1877) and The Principles of Light and Colour.

Most areas that seem to have been ignored in the past were emphasized by Edwin Babbitt. Babbitt presented a comprehensive theory of healing with colour. He identified the colour red as a stimulant, notably of blood and to a lesser extent the nerves; yellow and orange as nerve stimulants; blue and violet as soothing to all systems and as having anti-inflammatory properties.

Accordingly, Babbitt prescribed red for paralysis, physical exhaustion and chronic rheumatism; yellow as a laxative, emetic and purgative and for bronchial difficulties; blue for inflammatory conditions, sciatica, meningitis, nervous instability, headache, irritability and sunstroke. He also stated that 'all vital organs have direct connection with the skin through arteries, blood vessels and capillaries, and colour rays can affect the entire blood stream through circulation and elimination of toxins.

Babbitt also developed various devices, including a special cabinet called a thermolume, in which coloured glass and natural light were used to produce coloured light and a chrome disk—a funnel-shaped device fitted with a special colour filter—was used to focalize light onto various parts of the body.

He discussed in detail the effects of the reflection, absorption, transmission and polarization of light. Different patients were presented in his book who had been treated using colour healing devices created by him.

Babbitt also established the relationship between colour and minerals, which he used as an addition to treatment with coloured light, and he developed elixirs by irradiating water with sunlight filtered through coloured lenses. He claimed that this 'potentized water' retained the energy of the vital element within the particular colour filter used and had remarkable healing power. Babbitt was in fact among the pioneers of modern Chromotherapy. He used both direct and indirect methods of colour treatment. He seemed to be well aware of the techniques and methodologies used in Chromotherapy.

His invention of different devices such as a special cabinet that used natural light to produce coloured light by splitting it into seven colours, used for the focalization of light onto some particular area, worked quite effectively for healing wounds and stopping bleeding, headaches, etc. The actual energy to which he referred in potentized water was not calculated by any means. He did not explain the energy change in water, its quantum states and how different kinds of vibrations affect water in different manners. He did not explain about the potency of potentized water, but incredible for that time was his correlation of magnetism with Chromotherapy. His work on colour healing, for the first time in history, proved to be comprehensive in taking both a physiological and a psychological approach. Any chromotherapist even nowadays can benefit from his work as he discussed appropriate colours for diseases in detail that in a way does not contradict to the facts newly established under the influence of science.

In 1933, Indian-born American-citizen scientist Dinshah P. Ghadiali (1873-1966), referred to as the "Parsi Edison" published The Spectro Chromemetry Encyclopaedia, a work on Colour therapy. Ghadiali claimed to have discovered the scientific principles which explain why and how the different Coloured rays have various therapeutic effects on organisms. He believed that Colours represent chemical potencies in higher octaves of vibration, and for each organism and system of the body there is a particular Colour that stimulates and another that inhibits the work of that organ or system. Ghadiali also thought that by knowing the action of the different Colours upon the different organs and systems of the body, one can apply the correct Colour that will tend to balance the action of any organ or system that has become abnormal in its functioning or condition. Dinshah P. Ghadiali's son Darius Dinshah continues to provide information about Colour therapy via Dinshah Health Society, a nonprofit organization

He discovered the scientific principles that explain why and how different colour rays have various therapeutic effects on the body. His Spectro-Chrome Encyclopaedia, is considered to be the first published book to explain the complete doctrine of Chromotherapy. The rules explained in this book could be proved using any kind of modern techniques. Most chromopaths have used his technique.

He discovered that there is a unique colour or energy vibration that either sedates or stimulates the stream of energy through a specific organ, causing a natural biochemical reaction. By knowing the action of different colours upon the different organs and systems of the body, one can apply the appropriate colour that will balance the action of any organ or system that has become abnormal in its functioning or condition. When this balance is disturbed, mental and physical problems occur. The aim of the science of colour healing is to cure disease by restoring normal balance of colour energies of the body.

Ghadiali established that particular areas of the body respond to particular colours; these areas are similar to what the ancients called 'chakras'. According to Klotsche, 'the chakras are areas of highly concentrated energy that are connected to various locations mainly along the spinal cord. These energy fields are related to the major organs in the body. The concept of chakras is essentially an East Indian concept, which Ghadiali presented as the source of energies.

The work of Ghadiali actually demystified the theory of Chromotherapy. Ghadiali's research stated: 'The colour bands of spectrograms are produced when a chemical element undergoes a process of combustion or vaporization that accelerates the motion of its atoms. The specific band of colours and dark lines emitted when a certain element is heated, are known as Fraunhauafer lines. This procedure is commonly used to identify the chemical composition of a substance (with a photospectrometer).

Contrary to accepted scientific theory, which assumes that each element is a unit, Ghadiali concluded that 'the chemical elements are colour compounds'. His results can be proved by any of the sophisticated equipment of modern science. 'A specific disease thus constitutes a specific imbalance of colour waves and by implication, chemical imbalance.' Ghadiali found that by treating the body with a particular colour vibration, one could effectively reintroduce the appropriate biochemical elements into the body; he referred to this as colour chemistry, certainly a new field of study. His results as published in the first decade of the twentieth century were advocated by Klotsche in Colour Medicine: colour medicine not only can heal the diseased frequency of the body but also can introduce actual chemical elements/vibration into the body in a non-toxic form.

During the nineteenth century the emphasis in science was exclusively on matter rather than on energy. As medicine came under the umbrella of science, it focused too much on the material physical body, ignoring the mind. With the advances in physical medicine and treatments such as surgery and antiseptic, interest in healing with colours declined.

Throughout the 19th century "Colour healers" claimed Coloured glass filters could treat many diseases including constipation and meningitis.

A New Age conceptualisation of the chakras of Indian body culture and their positions in the human body
Practitioners of ayurvedic medicine believe the body has seven "chakras", which some claim are 'spiritual centers', and which are held to be located along the spine. New Age thought associates each of the chakras with a single Colour of the visible light spectrum, along with a function and organ or bodily system. According to this view, the chakras can become imbalanced and result in physical diseases, but application of the appropriate Colour can allegedly correct such imbalances.

P.V. Mihalache

Understanding Chakra and Colour Ray Frequency In 1951 Takkata discovered that 'Colour Ray Frequency changes in atmosphere arising from the sunspots really affect the flocculation index of human blood albumin resulting in changes of menstrual cycles.

Takkata came up with experimental results on direct exposure to sunlight. He did not mention anything about material aids for providing a colour deficient to the human body. Ott described Takkata's experiment in Part III of his series Colour and Light: Their Effect on Plants, Animals and People, published in 1987, and described how colour rays from sunspots would alter a person's flocculation index.

He further explained that there are different methods of applying coloured light. It can be received through the skin or the eyes, which, in turn, has been found to stimulate the internal glands. Ott's work seems to be a continuation of Takkata's efforts; both have worked on the effects of light on blood, but Ott also described the different methods of Chromotherapy. It is not clear in his work what parameters he has adopted to verify the effect of sunlight on skin. The same effect was also described in Babbitt's work, which is more informative and explanatory. It is very interesting that no chromopath has contradicted another's specific colour treatment suggested for a specific disease. Ott also emphasized the biological functioning of the human body when Chromotherapy is applied. He noted that different lights affect different enzymatic reactions for healing purpose. This was the first time that the effect of Chromotherapy was tested at the DNA level.

As Ghadiadi, Klotsche correlated colours with chakras:
Red   Root chakra
Orange Sacral chakra
Green   Heart chakra
Blue   Throat chakra
Indigo   Brow chakra
Violet   Crown chakra
White   Perfect colour blend

Each chakra energizes and sustains certain organs. The balance of the seven chakras activates healing by transmitting energy to the electromagnetic field around the body. The body has seven major energy centres known as chakras, each centres is responsive to a different colour. Chakra located at the sites of the major endocrine glands, corresponds to particular states of consciousness, personality types and endocrine secretions.

Approaches to Chromotherapy for new researchers, Klotsche discussed some useful points about Chromotherapy as he practiced it, and he found it to be a complete therapeutic system for 123 major illnesses. He used single colours and also combinations of two or more colours for therapy and different techniques, namely, direct exposure and hydrochromopathy. He correlated the concepts of colour healing with Einstein's mass–energy relationship, which seems quite accurate in terms of the concept of an energy field around the human body.

His work seems to be an extension of Ghadiali's concept, but it proved to be more accurate. He emphasized the pros of Chromotherapy—that it is safe, simple, economical and highly effective—but still his work lacks scientific proof on hydrochromopathy, which according to him was the best means of toxin elimination. We find no scientific calculations in his study; no spectroscopy has been conducted in this context.

Mester conducted experiments to determine the function of light in animal and human cells. The work of Mester resembles that of Azeemi and gives a clear picture of the effects of colours on the human body, whether applied directly to the skin or absorbed in such materials as water, oil and milk and then given to the patient. This could affect patients with hereditary diseases such as hypertension, thalassemia and diabetes. This work needs more research and a series of experiments should be carried out with certain biophysical applications.

Azeemi discussed in detail the causes of diseases and suggested appropriate colours, which are very easy to understand and to use.

He discussed in detail different methods of Chromotherapy but emphasized hydrochromopathy. The complete methodology of Chromotherapy as described by him is extremely useful and effective; undoubtedly, a new area of research has evolved with the publication of his book.

Hassan also adopted the methodology presented by Azeemi. His work is remarkable in the sense that he compiled all the concepts of chromopathy established so far.

Chromotherapists of the past emphasized one thing and left others unattended. Some have emphasized direct exposure of the affected and diseased area to light. Some have talked about the materials, and others have emphasized only watching colour. It is evident that all these methods focused only on the material aspect of Chromotherapy, but Hassan produced a detailed study covering different aspects of Chromotherapy, including the material aspect of healing as well as the electromagnetic transfer of colour characteristics. Hassan measured the production of a 32 su (sparkle units) charge in chromotized water due to the absorption of rays, but any theoretical explanation is missing. This was the first time in the history of Chromotherapy that this kind of work had been done, but surprisingly Hassan did not proceed further to the spectroscopy of charged water.

He also related seven musical tones to seven vibrational states and seven vitamins. He compared Chromotherapy with all other therapeutic systems developed so far, with an in-depth explanation of the complete doctrine of Chromotherapy (vibrational healing). He states: 'Every therapeutic system has its own doctrine or to say own point of view about the reasons and causes of diseases.' According to the theory of chromalux,

An electric charge is produced due to the influence of the vibrations of cosmic and colourful rays upon the brain cells. This electric charge takes the form of a current emitted where various cells collide with another.

This collision results in formation of incalculable colourful vibrations, which can be termed as thought.

The cervical vertebrae is the main passage for the current that starts from the brain; if this bone fractures, the flow of current suffers a setback resulting in damage of the brain tissues.

He elaborated the technique of choosing the right colour for specific diseases and explained the theory of the basic colours used for therapy and the combinations of different shades. Hassan's work stresses that a patient's history should be keenly observed before suggesting any colour.

Colour Psychology and Medicine For research techniques and impressive quantitative data, the world of colour psychology and medicine is indebted to the recent efforts of Gerard (1970). He painstakingly reviewed the whole area of light, colour and their psychophysiological influences. Probably for the first time, he tested the reactions of the entire organism, using advanced and modern techniques with coloured light beamed onto the skin of the subject. Profiting from the experience of other scientists and the use of an electroencephalogram, he evolved new approaches and discovered a number of significant facts.

Physiologically, affective responses of subjects revealed that warm colours were useful in arousing those troubled with reactive depression or neurasthenia. They increased muscle tone or blood pressure in hypertensive individuals. Cool colours elicited the reverse affective responses in all of the same tests.

Anxious subjects were actually calmed by these cooler colours, from the viewpoint of clinical psychology. This is an important finding in Gerard's work, as it reveals that cool colours can be effective as a tranquilizer in cases of tension and anxiety.

Physiologically, all colours produced clinically tangible results. Exposure to warm colours increased respiratory movements, frequency of eye blinks, cortical activation and palmar conductance (arousal of the autonomic nervous system).

Warm colours consistently showed a more pronounced pattern of stimulation. Cool colours showed opposite effects by acting as a relaxant and tranquilizer for anxious individuals, lowering blood pressure, providing relief from tension, alleviating of muscle spasms and reducing eye blink frequency. They also proved to be an aid for insomnia. Just as warm colours showed a consistently pronounced pattern of stimulation, cool colours showed a consistent pattern of relaxation. To summarize Gerard's research and testing, his scientific data showed that all colours affect all human both psychologically and physiologically in a specific manner.

Hassan related the human body to the electromagnetic energy glow surrounding every creature. In his view, this body or energy glow is responsible for keeping our body healthy. The same fact is described by Azeemi in his book Colour Therapy thus: 'It is a wrong concept that our physical body is itself everything, but instead the electromagnetic glow (aura) around the body gives us the energy and transfers health or diseases to the physical body'.

These concepts received support from Russian scientists who worked in collaboration with an Indian researcher, Shah, using Kirlian technology. They took pictures of the electromagnetic energy glow around the human body and discovered that actual disease appears first in the aura and is then transferred to our physical body and can be detected 6–8 months prior to appearance in our physical body. Thus, they have established the fact that Chromotherapy can be a preventive treatment.

In support of this theory, Thelma Moss noted: 'All seemingly solid objects in our world including our bodies are made up of the electromagnetic energy, the more dense the energy the more solid the object is.'

This fact also demonstrates an idea of Einstein's quoted by Shah in his article 'Divine healing', that if we are the objects with mass "m" and we expose ourselves to a very powerful and high intensity electromagnetic field, and then we will gradually be transformed from matter into energy.

In the form of energy, if we obtain a superior level of consciousness then we will be able to direct the flow of energy and we will not be restricted by the limited dimensions of space-time. Therefore in this condition we can surpass the boundary of time to return back into the past or to travel in the future. In addition to the fact that we are an energy source that possesses conscious wisdom, we have the capability to transform ourselves back to the physical form.

After Einstein's statement, a new door could be opened to justify the electromagnetic body around the physical body, as posited by Klotsche in Colour Medicine and that only Einstein could demonstrate to the materialistic or mechanized Newton-bound world of the West through his mathematical energy formula $E = mc2$.

According to Einstein energy and matter are interchangeable and interconvertible. Klotsche explains this phenomenon thus: We know that the vibratory rate of a substance determines its density or its forms as matter. When we recognize the vibratory patterns in the universe, i.e. the energy ranges or fields found on the cosmic electromagnetic scale, we will then be able to open the doors to the tremendous healing powers found in the subtle energy octaves of the cosmos. The visible light spectrum with its beneficial frequencies for the human body provides the preventing tool for healing. Colour Medicine is truly, the medicine of the future.

Chromotherapy provides colours to the electromagnetic body or the aura (energy field) around the body, which in turn transfers energy to the physical body. This makes Chromotherapy the most effective among various therapies.

When we speak of colour, we mean energy waves. Every colour, each with its own frequency, is a form of energy (12). Ghadiali agreed that beaming a colour or colours onto the skin acts as a form of feeding colour to the body. Patterson of Stellar Research Corporation explains that 'light is the closest thing to pure energy that we can identify.

Colour as pure vibrational energy is the rational therapy for maintaining health and overcoming disease. When applied to the human body, light will provide all deficient energies since every colour is associated with a quantity of energy. A concept from physics confirms the idea of chromotherapists that 'colours provide energies'. There have appeared no contradictions among any of the theories about Chromotherapy presented, but still there are some areas of study which were not focused on in the past, including the study of the electromagnetic radiation glow around the human body and its quantization.

Colours have a profound effect on us at all levels—physical, mental and emotional. If our energy levels are blocked or depleted, then our body cannot function properly, and this in turn can lead to a variety of problems at different levels.

This concept is also supported by Klotsche, who stated: These interrelating systems of subtle forces recharge or rechannel energy into diseased areas where it is blocked or deficient, for disease is nothing more than a restriction of energy flow. As we know energy or vibrational flow along the path of least resistance and through the extra energy associate with the use of vibrational healing, the appropriate energies seek out the needed areas, freeing blocked energy where it is most required.

The interaction between the dense physical energy of the body and the subtle energy, which controls many of the body functions or activities, is the key to understanding relationship between energy and matter.

This energy body can also be proved through photography, as described by Perry in scientific documentation of Chromotherapy: in 1939, Kirlian discovered that if an object on a photographic plate is subjected to a high voltage electric field, an image is created on the plate. The image looks like a coloured halo or a coronal discharge. This image is said to be the physical manifestation of the electromagnetic radiation around the body (aura), which allegedly surrounds every living thing.

Qalander explained unrevealed facts about the human body and its energy glow in his work. This idea has also been used by Shah and Russian medical staff for treating patients. This discovery led to a new area of research; unfortunately, scientists even today have not yet explored the relationship between the basic science of electromagnetic energy around the body (aura) and Chromotherapy.

Orthodox medicine and science give their own explanations of how light works. These explanations are based on strictly physical functions and ignore the bioelectric energy field, which has been demonstrated or photographed with Kirlian devices.

That electromagnetic energy can be moved through our auras into the physical body by light frequencies, using colour medicine, can also be explained thus: 'All living things are moist; the moisture is transferred from the subject to the emulsion to the electric charge pattern on the films, causing a Kirlian image to appear'. This undoubtedly helps us understand how disease is cured according to the doctrine of chromopathy, but the area that should be emphasized is the quantum state of electromagnetic radiance around every living body. Variation in Influences of Light During the 1950s, studies suggested that neonatal jaundice, a potentially fatal condition found in two-thirds of premature babies, could be successfully treated by exposure to sunlight.

This was confirmed in the 1960s, and white light replaced high-risk blood transfusions in the treatment of this condition. Blue light was later found to be more effective and less hazardous than full-spectrum light (the most common form of treatment for neonatal jaundice). Comparison of blue light with turquoise for treatment of neonatal jaundice was carried out by Ebbesen. Bright white full-spectrum light is also now being used in the treatment of cancers, SAD (seasonal affective disorder, so-called winter depression), anorexia, bulimia nervosa, insomnia, jetlag, shift working, alcohol and drug dependency, and to reduce overall levels of medication.

Schauss worked on the tranquilizing effect of colours and found that colour reduces aggressive behavior and violence.

The blue light found to be successful in the treatment of neonatal jaundice has also been shown to be effective in the treatment of rheumatoid arthritis, as emphasized by Pleasanton in his work. In studies by McDonald, most of those exposed to blue light for variable periods of up to 15 min experienced a significant degree of pain relief. It was concluded that the pain reduction was directly related both to the blue light and to the length of exposure to it.

Blue light is also used in healing injured tissue and preventing scar tissue, as well as for burns and lung conditions. In 1990, scientists reported to the annual conference of the American Association for the Advancement of Science on the successful use of blue light in the treatment of a wide variety of psychological problems, including addictions, eating disorders and depression.

At the other end of the colour spectrum, red light has been shown to be effective in the treatment of cancer and constipation and in healing wounds. As a result, colour is becoming widely accepted as a therapeutic tool with various medical applications.

A new technique that has been developed over the past two decades as a result of pioneering research is photodynamic therapy (PDT).

This is based on the discovery that certain intravenously injected photosensitive chemicals not only accumulate in cancer cells but also selectively identify these cells under ultraviolet light.

These photosensitive chemicals then exclusively destroy the cancer cells when activated by red light, whose longer wavelength allows it to penetrate tissue more deeply than other colours.

PDT can be used for both diagnosis and treatment. Thomas Dougherty, who developed PDT, reports that in a worldwide experiment more than 3000 people with a wide variety of malignant tumors have been successfully treated using this.

Chromotherapy is now used to improve the performance of athletes; whereas red light appears to help athletes who need short, quick bursts of energy, blue light assists in performances requiring a steadier energy output.

By comparison, pink light has a tranquilizing and calming effect within minutes of exposure. It suppresses hostile, aggressive and anxious behavior. Pink holding cells are now widely used to reduce violent and aggressive behavior among prisoners, and some sources have reported a reduction of muscle strength in inmates within 2.7 s. It appears that when in pink surroundings people can never become aggressive despite their desire, because the colour saps their energy. In contrast, yellow should be avoided in such contexts because it is highly stimulating. Gimbel suggested a possible relationship between violent street crime and sodium yellow street lighting.

Colour, Brain and the Effects of Light Research in Russia during the 1960s showed that one in six experimental subjects could recognize colour with their fingertips after only 20–30 min training, and blind people developed this sensitivity even more quickly. Understanding of these effects has come about only as a result of research into the hormones melatonin and serotonin, both of which are produced by the pineal gland in the brain.

P.V. Mihalache

Melatonin is known to be the crucial chemical pathway by which animals respond to light and synchronize their bodily functioning with diurnal and seasonal variations. Serotonin is a very important neurotransmitter in the brain, whose action has been linked with mental disturbances such as schizophrenia and hallucinogenic states. Serotonin, a stimulant, is produced during daylight whereas the output of melatonin – which is linked with sleep – increases when it is dark and has a generally depressive effect. This is reversed when it is light and the production of melatonin drops. Its main site of action appears to be the hypothalamus, the part of the brain involved in mediating the effects of various hormones and in regulating emotions.

However, changes in the output of melatonin in response to light influence every cell of the body, notably the reproductive processes, which are sensitive to such variations. High levels of melatonin have been found in women with ovulation problems and anorexia nervosa (a characteristic feature of which is amenorrhea, or absence of periods), in men with low sperm count and in people suffering from SAD, which usually occurs during winter.

Research also confirmed that certain parts of the brain are not only light sensitive but actually respond differently to different wavelengths; it is now believed that different wavelengths (colours) of radiation interact differently with the endocrine system to stimulate or reduce hormone production..

This work has given a new dimension to Chromotherapy: the use of colours in psychological disorders. SAD has become a very common problem nowadays, in England in particular, where the sun does not shine for up to 1 or 2 weeks, so that no light enters into the body. As a consequence, psychological diseases manifest, mainly in the form of depressions, which, according to chromopathy studies, are curable without any use of tranquilizers.

A detailed study of Chromotherapy, with patients exposed to sunlight through colour filters, was produced by Jacob. He adopted modern theories to prove the relationship between melatonin, light and colour.

Takkata was the first researcher to attempt to find a relationship between blood and sunlight. Jacob's work concerns hormonal changes as a result of exposure to sunlight. Of course, sunlight is a perfect blend of seven colours; different colours are responsible for the release of different kinds of hormones, which keeps us healthy. Jacob stated in his work that

Light is responsible for turning on the brain and the body. Light enters the body through the eyes and skin. When even a single photon of light enters the eye, it lights up the entire brain.

This light triggers the hypothalamus, which regulates all life-sustaining bodily functions, the autonomic nervous system, endocrine system, and the pituitary (the body's master gland).

The hypothalamus is also responsible for our body's biological clock. It also sends a message, by way of light, to the pineal organ, which is responsible for releasing one of our most important hormones, melatonin. The release of melatonin is directly related to light, darkness, colours, and the Earth's electromagnetic field. This necessary hormone affects every cell in the body. It turns on each cell's internal activities, allowing them to harmonize with each other and nature.

The pineal gland is believed to be responsible for our feeling of oneness with the universe and sets the stage for the relationship between our inner being and the environment. If that relationship is harmonious, we are healthy, happy, and feel a sense of well-being. An imbalance in this relationship makes itself known in the form of disorders or disease in our physical, mental or emotional states.

The Pineal is our "light meter", and receives information from the heavens above, to give us that sense of oneness with the universe, and from the Earth's electromagnetic field below to keep us grounded. A perfect balance is necessary to maintain our health and to keep us in harmony with the environment.

Many aspects of humankind's explorations are ignored, neglected or discarded. Colour medicine is one of these neglected items.

The common feature of every remedial and curative system of treatment, whether it is Ayurveda, allopathy, acupuncture, Unani, homeopathy, biochemic, magnetotherapy, physiotherapy, radiotherapy, aromatherapy, reflexology or Chromotherapy, is to somehow apply vibrations of one kind or another in such a manner that the body can be put back on the health track.

Most systems induce vibrations indirectly, but there are a few in which the vibrations are used directly upon the body, and Chromotherapy is one of them.

Babbitt, Ghadiali and Azeemi revolutionized to the development of Chromotherapy. Their ideas were carried out by other researchers. No controversies were found among the theories presented, in research work conducted in any area of the world.

We conjecture that colour is a quantum state of matter. There are other quantum states such as charm, beauty, flavor, tenderness, etc. These quantum states are linked with each other via 'glucons' and form intermediatory energy fields known as 'quarks'.

Quarks, if condensed, produce bosons, a fifth state of matter. The medium used in Chromotherapy has never been explored in depth; for example, water, the main medium used in Chromotherapy, has never been studied quantitatively in any of the research conducted in the context of Chromotherapy. The literature exhibits a severe lack of scientific work pertaining to quantum physical states and optical mathematics.

Similarly no proofs available on the basis of scientific calculations of chromotized water. We found no study of quantum states and the electromagnetic glow around the human body. Conductivity measurements of the chromotized water used in hydrochromopathy have not been emphasized by any researcher.

Mass–energy-related measurements could be helpful in potentizing or chromotizing the liquid medium used for treatment. Relationships ought to be established between charged water, its energy states and its effect on the human body. The quantum mechanical dipole moment as a result of absorption of different colours, we conjecture, produces charge quantization phenomena. Chromotherapy as a system of treatment can benefit people because of its harmony with nature. Everything that exists in this world is a combination of different colours . In every creation of God, one colour or another is dominant; as stated by Azeemi:

By using clay, a clay pot is repaired and piece of cloth mends a doll made of cloth, the plastic is used to repair the articles of plastic, then why light and colours cannot be used for the human health care which is the origin of man's creation. The holy scriptures say that existence of man is based upon various types of lights and colours. Then why a human being cannot be treated with colours.

Walker once said: You realize you are part of the hologram of life, surrounded by an aura or energy field that radiates distinct colour and vibrations. The aura fingertips your soul and reflects your goodness, wellness, mental stability, maturity, emotional/inner turmoil or peaceful fulfilment. More of each of these qualities, peace, wellness, stability, maturity and fulfilment may become your ever present precious possession by the application of colour's power in our daily living.

3. HOW COLOURS AFFECT US

A preference for certain colours can point at two simple things:

- self-expression - you choose the colours which match your personality; for instance green for a lover of harmony and nature
- completion - you choose the colours you need more of; for instance an active, passionate person chooses blue colours to cool down his nature.

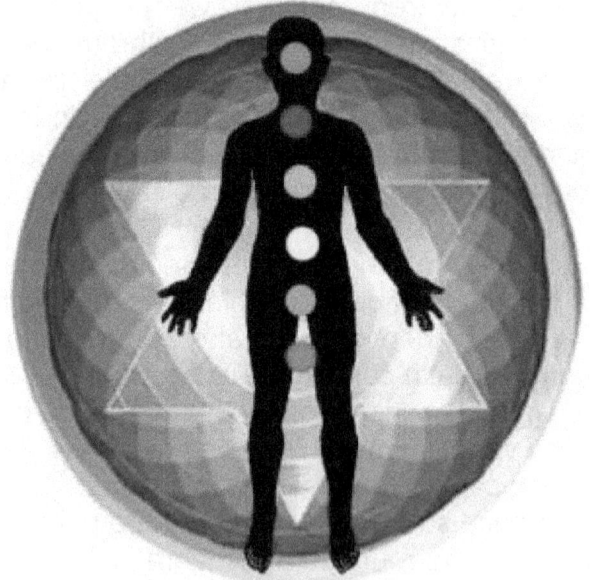

An aversion against certain colours gives information as well.

Black is a powerful, mysterious colour and is associated with seriousness. Also associated with sex, death and mystery. Black may make you feel depressed, or on the other hand, may make you feel secure - "hiding in the darkness."

Blue is a relaxing colour. Blue lowers blood pressure, calms, gives a sense of security, and suppresses appetite.

Brown is an organic, earthy colour. It can make you feel cozy.

Green is the easiest colour for the eyes to focus on for long periods of time. It soothes pain and is associated with optimism. May make one feel happy, clean, fresh.

Orange colour is friendly, relaxing and ambitious.

Pink is a youthful, feminine colour. Pink is also a soft, sensitive colour. This is basically a "happy" colour.

Purple colour is often associated with royalty. It is also a contemporary colour. Purple has a list of associated feelings, from feeling mournful to creative.

Red colour raises the blood pressure, stimulates appetite and conversation and is often associated with excitement, action, impulse.

White is often associated with purity, cleanliness. Also associated with nothingness, and in some cultures death and/or mourning. Can make one feel clean/sterile

Yellow is an eye irritant and a highly emotional colour.

After long periods of time, yellow invokes feelings of anger and hostility. However, in small doses, is a friendly, happy colour.

Red

Red is associated with the base chakra in the sacral region. It promotes vitality, strength, sexuality, willpower, and alertness. Red is used to counteract anemia, lack of energy, impotence, and low blood pressure. Its complement is turquoise.

The key features or red colour are: Strengthening of the life force, will and sexuality.

Physical:

- Red is the element of fire. Red rays produce heat which vitalizes and energizes the physical body.
- Red stimulates and excites the nerves and the blood.
- Red stimulates the sensory nerves. It is beneficial in deficiencies of smell, sight, hearing, taste and touch.
- Red activates the circulation of the blood, excites the cerebro-spinal fluid and sympathetic nervous systems.
- Red is good for the muscular system and the left cerebral brain hemisphere. It is excellent for contracted muscles.
- Red builds the hemoglobin. It energizes the liver.
- Red rays decompose the salt crystals in the body and act as a catalyst for ionization.
- Red is particularly useful in the absorption of iron into the body.
- Red clears congestion and the mucous.
- Red affects the circulatory system and sexuality. It stimulates the overall energy levels of the metabolism, lower extremities and most blood conditions.
- Red is a stimulating colour. It will energize the base chakra. It warms and it activates. It awakens our physical life force.

Psychological
- Red represents health, fire, anger, temper, danger and destruction.
- Red stimulates, excites, and acts as an irritant.
- Red gives the person a sense of power.
- Red is helpful for the presbyopic or far-sighted individual to become ego-centered.
- Red draws the ego back into the self.
- Red is used for the extrovert to go back into his shell.

Red may be useful for colds, poor circulation, anemia, and mucus ailments. Red strengthens the physical energy and the will of the individual. It can stimulate deeper passions, whether they are of sex and love, courage, hatred or even revenge.

Red May Be useful in the Treatment of :
- Anemia
- Blood ailments
- Bronchial Asthma
- Bronchitis
- Constipation
- Endocrine System- Red is useful in the management of stress. It also plays a key role in the health of the individual-physically, mentally, emotionally, and spiritually
- Listlessness
- Melancholia
- Paralysis
- Physical Debility
- Pneumonia
- Tuberculosis

Do Not Use Red In Case of :
- Emotionally disturbed people
- Excitable temperaments
- Fever
- Florid complexioned people
- Hypertension

- Inflammatory conditions
- Insanity - Avoid red in most cases of insanity and emotional disturbances.
- Neuritis
- Red-Headed individuals

Excessive use of red will produce fever and exhaustion. It promotes hostility, anger, violence. Too much red can over-stimulate and aggravate certain conditions. High blood pressure is an indication of too much red energy within the system. It is recommended that red be used in conjunction with blue rays. Red is balanced by the colour green

Healing properties: Brings warmth, energy and stimulation, therefore good for energy, fatigue, colds, chilly and passive people. Red energizes heart and blood circulation, it builds up the blood and heightens a low blood pressure. Energizes all organs and the senses hearing, smell, taste, vision and touch. Increases sexual desire and activity. Stimulates ovulation and menstruation.

Red links with and stimulates the root chakra, at the base of the spine, causing the adrenal glands to release adrenalin. This results in greater strength. Red causes hemoglobin to multiply, thus increasing energy and raising body temperature. It is excellent for anemia and blood-related conditions. It loosens, opens up clogs, releases stiffness and constrictions. It is excellent for areas that have become stiffened or constricted.

Esoteric/magical: Deities of love, passion, sexuality and war. Great energy, courage, will-power, determination, speed, assertiveness, aggression, masculinity, independence, physical strength, sports, competition, conflicts, health, sexual attraction and potency, love and passion, fertility.

Preference for red: Red is associated with passionate love, sex, great energy, impulse, action and stimulation, assertiveness and aggression, courage, strength and power, adventure, danger, warnings, revolt and revolution.

Temperamental and ambitious people with a need for personal freedom.

Aversion to red: A person who has an aversion to red may be over-active, too impulsive, hot-tempered, aggressive and egocentric, or have difficulties with people with such characteristics. It can also symbolize deeply hidden fears and rejection of his own assertiveness.

Orange

Orange is associated with the spleen chakra, which regulates circulation and metabolism. Orange stimulates the thyroid gland, is a respiratory stimulant, but a depressant of parathyroid action. The orange vibration expands the lungs. Orange promotes happiness and joyousness. Orange is used to treat depression, hypothyroidism and kidney and lung problems, such as asthma and bronchitis. Its complement is blue.

The Key Features of Orange are activation, construction, optimism and building up energy reserves.

Physical:

- Orange has an antispasmatic effect. It is useful for muscle spasms or cramps of all kinds.
- Orange acts on the spleen and the pancreas to help assimilation and circulation. It aids the calcium metabolism of the body and strengthens the lungs.
- Orange stimulates the milk producing action of the breast after child birth.
- Orange stimulates and increases the pulse rate without affecting the blood pressure.

Psychological:

- Orange combines physical energy with mental qualities.
- Orange releases the energy from both chakras of the spleen and the pancreas.

- Orange is the colour for ideas and mental concepts.
- Orange strengthens the etheric body, enlivens the emotions, and creates a general sense of well-being and cheerfulness.
- Orange symbolizes warmth and prosperity.
- Orange is the colour of heat, fire, will, and temporal power.
- Orange affects the second (spleen) chakra center. It is the colour of joy and wisdom and creativity.
- Orange stimulates feelings of socialness.
- Orange is tied to our emotional health and the muscular system of the body.

Orange can assist us in healing conditions of the spleen, pancreas, stomach, intestines, adrenals, food assimilation, and depression.

Individuals experiencing emotional paralysis can be helped with this colour, especially the peach shades. Peach is a colour that strengthens the aura and gives it a little extra cushioning in recovery processes. It and most shades of orange can be used to revitalize the physical body. It makes a good tonic after a bout of illness, for it is strengthening to the eliminative system of the body.

Diseases Treated with Orange:

- Asthma
- Bronchitis
- Colds
- Epilepsy
- Gall stones
- Gout
- Growths-malignant and non-malignant.
- Hyper-Hypothyroidism
- Lung condition
- Malignancy
- Mestruation-cessation
- Mental exhaustion
- Kidney ailments

- Prolapsus
- Tumors
- Rheumatism

Too much orange may adversely affects the nerves. It can also aggravate the second or sex chakra. Orange should be balanced with shades of green-blues.

Healing properties: Orange is warm, cheering, non-constricting. Orange has a freeing action upon the body and mind, relieving repressions.

Orange shows new possibilities and other options in life. Stimulates creative thinking and enthusiasm, and helps assimilate new ideas. It is also helpful in dealing with excess sexual expression.

Orange stimulates the lungs, the respiration and the digestion. Increases the activity of the thyroid. Reliefs muscle cramps and spasms. Increases the amount of mother milk.

Finally, orange links very strongly with the sacral chakra.

Esoteric/magical: Deities of good luck and fortune. Attraction, charm, kindness, encouragement, stimulation, optimism, success, abundance, prosperity, feast and celebration, energy, achieving business-goals, investments, success in legal matters.

Preference for orange: Orange represents the warmth of the fire. It brings even more energy than yellow, celebration and great abundance, comfort, enjoyment of the senses. Warm, sociable, dynamic and independent people who dedicate themselves to whatever they do.

Aversion to orange: A person who has an aversion to orange may have suppressed sexual feelings or other difficulties with sensual enjoyment of life.

The attitude can also be over-sensual, indulgent, or too materialistic.

Yellow

Yellow is associated with the solar plexus chakra, which is concerned with intellect and judgment.

Yellow stimulates mental ability and concentration, and aids detachment. It can be used to treat rheumatism and arthritis, as well as straw related illnesses. Its complement is violet.

Key Features of the Yellow colour includes strong mental activity, intellectual power and ability, awakening

Physical:

- Yellow activates the motor nerves. It generates energy for the muscles. Disturbance in the supply of yellow energy to any part of the body can cause disturbance of function in that area including partial or complete paralysis from the deficiency of sensory and/or motor energy.
- Yellow affects the digestive system, gastrointestinal tract, adrenal activity and the left hemisphere brain activity.
- Yellow is excellent for the nerves and the brain; It is a motor stimulant and a nerve builder.
- Yellow rays strengthen the nerves and aid the brain.
- Yellow has a stimulating, cleansing, and eliminating action on the liver, intestines, and the skin.
- Yellow purifies the blood stream. It activates the lymphatic system.
- Yellow is a spleen depressant, cathartic, cholegogue, antheimintic.

Psychological:

- Yellow is good for despondent and melancholy conditions.
- To the ancients, yellow was the animating colour for life; it suggests joy, gaiety, merriment.
- Yellow is the colour of the intellect, of perception rather than of reason.

- The golden-yellow shades are healthful to both the body and the mind. It can be used to facilitate the learning capabilities of an individual.
- Yellow is a colour that catches the eye. It is one of the first colours that most people notice. It is also a colour that can create or indicate anxiety and mental tension.

Yellow is a mixture of red and green rays. It has half the stimulating potency of red and half the reparative potency of the green. Hence, it tends both to stimulate function and to repair damaged cells. Yellow light directed at the intestinal tract for short periods is a digestant. For longer periods, it acts both as catharsis and as a cathartic. It also stimulates the flow of bile and has an anthelmintic action becoming antagonistic to parasites and worms.

Yellow predominantly affects the solar plexus chakra, and it is stimulating to the mental faculties of the individual. It can be used for depression. It helps awaken an enthusiasm for life. It awakens greater confidence and optimism. It is also effective in the treatment of digestive problems. It is beneficial to the stomach, the intestines, the bladder, and the entire eliminative system as well. It is very effective in the treatment of most headaches. It helps to balance the gastrointestinal tract.

Diseases treated with Yellow:
- Constipation
- Diabetes
- Digestive Processes
- Eczema
- Flatulence
- Hemiplegic
- Kidney problems
- Indigestion
- Liver problems
- Mental/depression and exhaustion
- Paralysis
- Rheumatism

Does Not Use Yellow If You Are Suffering From:
- Acute inflammation
- Delirium
- Diarrhea
- Fever
- Neuralgia
- Over-Excitement
- Palpitation of the heart

Excessive amounts or exposures to yellow may make one superficial or hyperactive. It should be balanced with colours from the blue spectrum.

Healing properties: Yellow helps strengthen the nerves and the mind. It helps awaken mental inspiration and stimulates higher mentality. Thus, it is an excellent colour for nervous or nerve-related conditions or ailments. It also energizes the muscles. Dark yellow soothes pains in the nerves , also known as shooting pains.

Yellow can be used for conditions of the stomach, liver, and intestines. Speeds up the digestion and assimilation, and the stool. It helps the pores of the skin and aids scarred tissue in healing itself.

Yellow links with and stimulates the solar plexus, or psychic center. It can be used for psychic burnout or other psychic-related conditions or ailments. Activates and cheers up depressed and melancholic people. Gives lust for life.

Esoteric/magical: Elemental air. Deities for trade, travel, knowledge and magic. Life-force, vitality, change, progress, contact, communication, trade, commerce, to persuade with confidence, joy, cheerfulness, learning, knowledge, mental clarity, concentration, memorizing, tests, speaking and writing, traveling, affirmation, visualization.

Preference for yellow: The colour of the sun, life-force, vividity, vitality and energy. The colour of cheerfulness, curiosity, alternation, flexibility, progress, amusement, contact through traveling and communication, learning and practical knowledge. A feeling for writing and speaking.

Aversion to yellow: A person who has aversion to yellow may be emotionally disappointed and bitter.

May have tendency to rationalize feelings, or to avoid the depth of life by often changing relationships, many superficial relationships and/or constant changing activities.

Green

Green is the colour of the heart chakra. Green is the colour of nature. Green is the most predominant colour on the planet. It balances our energies, and it can be used to increase our sensitivity and compassion. It represents purity and harmony.

It has a calming effect, especially in inflamed conditions of the body. It is soothing to the nervous system. It is a great healer. It builds muscles, bones and other tissue cells. Its complement is magenta.

The key features of green are balance, growth, calming.
Physical:

- Green is cooling, soothing, and calming both physically and mentally. If you are exhausted, green initially has a beneficial effect, but after a time, it becomes tiring.
- Green acts upon the sympathetic nervous system. It relieves tension in the blood vessels and lowers the blood pressure. It acts upon the nervous system as a sedative and is helpful in sleeplessness, exhaustion, and irritability.
- Green dilates the capillaries and produces a sensation of warmth.
- Green is a muscle and tissue builder.
- Green is an aphrodisiac and a sex tonic.
- Green is a disinfectant, germicide, antiseptic and bacteriocide.

Psychological:
- Green awakens greater friendliness, hope, faith, and peace.
- Green is restful and revitalizing to overtaxed mental conditions. It is emotionally soothing.
- Green loosens and equalizes the etheric body.
- Green is the colour of energy, youth, growth, inexperience, fertility, hope, and new life.
- Green is the colour of envy, jealousy, and superstition.
- Green is an emotional stabilizer and pituitary stimulant.

Green strongly affects the heart chakra, and it is balancing to the autonomic nervous system. It can be applied beneficially in cardiac conditions, high blood pressure, ulcers, exhaustion, and headaches.

Green harmonizes, life-giving, calms the mind, nerves, fever, and acidity; balances the metabolism, stabilizes the weight, tones liver and spleen; and benefits the pituitary gland.

Diseases Treated with Green:
- Asthma
- Back disorders- small and lower back
- Cold
- Colic
- Erysipelas
- Exhaustion
- Hay fever
- Heart conditions
- Hepatic ailments
- High blood pressure
- Irritability
- Laryngitis
- Malaria
- Malignancy
- Nervous system

- Nervous diseases

- Neuralgia
- Overstimulation
- Piles
- Sleeplessness
- Syphilis
- Typhoid
- Ulcers
- Venereal diseases

Green should never be used to help heal tumorous or cancerous conditions or with anything of a malignant nature as green helps things grow.

Healing properties: Green is the colour of Nature and the earth. It is balance and harmony in essence and possesses a soothing influence upon both mind and body. It is neither relaxing nor astringent in its impact.

Green can be used for just about any condition in need of healing. Green rings psychological and emotional harmony and balance.

Green links with and stimulates the heart chakra. Green affects blood pressure and all conditions of the heart. It has both an energizing effect and a moderating or soothing effect.

It cures hormonal imbalances. Stimulates growth hormone and rejuvenation. Cleans and purifies from germs, bacteria and rotting material. Harmonizes the digestion, stomach, liver, gall.

Has a healing effect on kidneys. Increases immunity. Builds up muscles, bones and tissues. Stimulates inner peace. Strengthens the nervous system.

Esoteric/magical: Elemental earth (dark green) and elemental water (blue-green). Nature, fertility, growth, rejuvenation, recovering, healing, harvest and abundance, prosperity, harmony, balance, peace, hope, mother earth, home, herbal magic, plants and animals, counteract greed and jealousy.

Preference for green: Green brings peace, rest, hope,

comfort and nurturing, calmness and harmony.

Interest in nature, plants, fellowmen, children and animals, health and healing, natural and plain life. Longing for a safe home and family-life. A dislike of conflicts.

Aversion to green: A person who has an aversion to green may be more interested in independence and self-development than in a warm family-life. May prefer to keep a certain distance in (sexual) relationships.

Blue

Blue is associated with the throat chakra, which deals with willpower and communication. Blue is a calming colour, good for curing insomnia. It can be used for throat problems, asthma, stress, and migraine, and it is good for improving verbal skills. Its complement is orange.

The Key Features of Blue are peace, faith, aspiration, creative expression

Physical:

- Blue stimulates metabolism and builds vitality.
- Blue promotes growth.
- Blue slows the action of the heart and are therefore good for tachycardia.
- Blue has a tonic effect.
- Blue has antiseptic properties and is bacteriocidal.
- Blue is cold, electrical, and has contracting potencies.
- Blue contracts the arteries, veins, and capillaries and thereby raises the blood pressure.
- Blue is anticarcinogenic.
- Blue is excellent for inflammatory diseases. It has a soothing and cooling effect on them.
- Blue reduces nervous excitement.
- Blue is cooling, soothing, and astringent.

Psychological:

- Blue is good for over-excitement.

- Blue is used for the introvert to come out of his shell
- Blue is good in cases of the manic depressive-for the manic phase
- Blue is more soothing than green in emotional conditions.
- Blue is the colour for meditation and spiritual expansion.
- Blue relaxes the mind and controls the throat chakra, which is the creative power center.
- Blue is helpful in myopia physically and psychologically for it draws the ego outward, making the individual field oriented and more in harmony with his environment.
- Prolonged exposure, more than 10 minutes, to blue rays may make people feel tired and begin to feel depressed. Blue clothing and blue furnishings if not broken up with other colours make one tired and depressed.
- Blue is the colour for truth, devotion, calmness, and sincerity.
- Blue is the colour of intuition and the higher mental faculties.
- Blue promotes solitude, meditation, and independence.

Blue is cooling to the body's system. It is relaxing. It is quieting to our energies, and it has an antiseptic effect. It strengthens and balances the respiratory system. It is also excellent for high blood pressure and all conditions of the throat. It is beneficial to venous conditions of the body.

Blue is very effective in easing all childhood diseases, along with asthma, chicken pox, jaundice, and rheumatism. It is one of the most universally heating colours for children. It can also be used to awaken intuition and to ease loneliness. It awakens artistic expression and inspiration.

Blue helps reduce tumors, congestion, fevers, and infections; neutralizes anger and hatred; cools the mind and eyes, eyes and the pineal gland.

Diseases Treated with Blue:
- Apoplexy
- Baldness
- Biliousness
- Bowels
- Bums
- Cataracts
- Chicken pox
- Cholera
- Colic
- Diarrhea
- Dysentery
- Eye-inflammation
- Epilepsy
- Febrile diseases
- Gastro-Intestinal disease
- Hydrophobia
- Hysteria
- Insomnia
- Itching
- Jaundice
- Laryngitis
- Measles
- Menstruation-pain
- Palpitation
- Polio
- Glaucoma
- Gonorrhea
- Headache
- Renal Diseases
- Rheumatism-acute Scarlet fever
- Shock
- Syphilis
- Throat trouble-all tonsillitis
- Typhoid Fever

- Ulcers: Duodenal
- Gastric problems
- Vomiting
- Whooping cough

Do Not Use Blue If You Are Suffering From:

- Colds
- Constriction of muscles
- Hypertension
- Muscles-constriction
- Paralysis
- Rheumatism-chronic
- Tachycardia

Excess blue can make one overly cold-natured.

Healing properties: Blue is cooling, electric, astringent. Dr. Edwin Babbitt, in his classic, "The Principles of Light and Colour," states that "The Blue Ray is one of the greatest antiseptics in the world."

Cools down inflammations even rheumatic inflammations, fever, high blood pressure, stops bleedings, reliefs the bursting headaches, calms strong emotions like anger, aggression or hysteria. Brings tranquility. Anti-itching. Anti-irritation, for instance redness of the skin, anti-stress. Soothes suffering.

Blue can be used for any type of ailments associated with speech, communication, or the throat. Excellent for laryngitis or inflammation of the larynx.

Blue links with and stimulates the throat chakra. The throat chakra is often referenced as the "power center" and "the greatest center in the body" because it is the primary center of expression and communication, through speech.

Esoteric/magical: Elemental water and elemental air. Deities of the sea, truth and wisdom. Peace and tranquility, calmness, truth, wisdom, justice, counsel, guidance, understanding, patience, loyalty and honor, sincerity, devotion, healing, femininity, prophetic dreams, protection during sleep, astral projection.

Preference for blue: Cool and soothing, dreamy and magical. Peace and rest. For people who keep a certain distance, but give calm and practical help; they are faithful and loyal, have a sense for order, logic and rational thinking. Flying in day-dreaming, ideals or nostalgia when felt miss-understood. Dark blue is more severe and can be melancholic. Blue is also the colour of truth.

Aversion to blue: A person who has an aversion to blue, may be very disciplined, strong career worker, with an aversion of commentary or restriction. He may have charted out a clear direction for his life and wants to follow that lacelike .

Indigo

Indigo and the deeper shades of blue are dynamic healing colours on both spiritual and physical levels. Indigo is balancing to all conditions associated with it. It strengthens the lymph system, the glands, and the immune system of the body. It is an excellent blood purifier, and can be used to assist in detoxifying the body.

The Key Characteristics are integration, purification, altered states of consciousness

Physical:

- Indigo is electric, cooling and astringent.
- Indigo stimulates the parathyroid and depresses the thyroid.
- Indigo is a purifier of the blood stream.
- Indigo helps reduce or stop excessive bleeding.
- Indigo is good for muscular tonicity.
- Indigo is a respiratory depressor.
- Indigo can be effective as an anesthetic and can induce total insensibility.

The patients become insensible to pain without losing consciousness after being exposed to indigo. It seems to raise the consciousness of the patient to such a high level of vibration that he/she becomes unaware of the physical body.

Psychological
- Indigo controls the psychic currents of the subtle bodies.
- Indigo governs the chakra that controls the pineal gland.
- Indigo has a sedative effect, and it can be used in meditation to achieve deeper levels of consciousness.
- Indigo can awaken devotion and intuition.
- Indigo affects vision, hearing, and smell on the physical, emotional, and spiritual plane.

Indigo can be used effectively to treat all conditions of the face including the eyes, ears, nose, mouth, and sinuses. It can be used for problems in the lungs and for removing obsessions.

Diseases Treated with Indigo:
- Appendicitis
- Asthma
- Bronchitis
- Cataracts
- Convulsions
- Delirium Tremens or Delirium Tremors
- Dyspepsia
- Ear-deafness
- Ear difficulties
- Ear diseases - abnormal sounds in the ear
- Eye diseases
- Hyperthyroidism
- Insanity
- Lung trouble
- Nervous ailments
- Nasal diseases
- Nose Bleed
- Nose ailments

- Obsession
- Palsy
- Paralysis-facial
- Pneumonia
- Smell problems
- Throat diseases
- Tonsillitis
- Whooping cough

Too much indigo can cause depression and a sense of separateness from others. It can be balanced effectively with soft orange shades.

Healing properties: Indigo is a great purifier of the bloodstream and also benefits mental problems. It is a freeing and purifying agent.

Indigo combines the deep blue of devotion with a trace of stabilizing and objective red. Indigo is cool, electric, and astringent. Indigo links with and stimulates the brow chakra - the third eye - and controls the pineal gland. It governs both physical and spiritual perception.

It can be of great assistance in dealing with ailments of the eyes and ears.

Violet

Violet is the colour of the crown chakra, which is concerned with the energy of the higher mind. It also affects the entire skeletal and nervous systems of the body.

It is very antiseptic, purifying on both physical and spiritual levels. It helps balance the physical and the spiritual energies. Violet is effective in cancerous conditions of the body. Arthritis can be eased by a violet light that leans more toward the blue shades. Violet also helps the body assimilate nutrients and minerals. It is the colour of dignity, honor, self-respect, and hope. It is used to bolster self-esteem and counter feelings of hopelessness, as well as in the treatment of mental and nervous disorders.

Key characteristics are purification, transmutation, practical spirituality. Its complement is yellow.

Physical

- Violet stimulates the spleen.
- Violet depresses the motor nerve, lymphatic and cardiac systems
- Violet nourishes the blood in the upper brain. It purifies the blood.
- Violet maintains the potassium and sodium balance of the body
- Violet is good for bone-growth.

Psychological

- Violet stimulates inspiration and humility. It assists in stimulating dream activity.
- A true violet is fifty percent blue and fifty percent red. It is the balance of the physical and the spiritual. It is a reminder that we need both aspects within our life for balanced health. Violet helps to restore a proper perspective both in regard to the mundane aspects of life (including the physical well-being), and the spiritual aspects, helping to keep them practical.
- Violet is excellent in calming or overcoming the excesses of violent insanity. It controls irritability in the sane. Violet controls excess hunger.
- Violet is an inspiring and spiritual colour. In meditation violet can help open us to our past lives, especially those which are presently affecting our health. Leonardo da Vinci believed that the power of meditation can be magnified ten-fold under the violet light falling through the stained glass window of a quiet church.
- Violet is a healing colour. Violet is the ruler of the center of the head called the Thousand- Petalled Lotus.

Diseases Treated with Violet:
- Bladder trouble
- Bone growth
- Cerebro spinal meningitis
- Concussion
- Cramps
- Epilepsy
- Kidneys
- Leucoderma
- Mental disorders
- Neuralgia
- Nervous disorders
- Rheumatism
- Sciatica
- Scalp diseases
- Skin
- Tumors
- Precautions

May stagnate or suppress emotions - especially anger.

Healing properties is the colour of transformation. It heal melancholy, hysteria, delusions and alcohol addiction and bring spiritual insights and renewal. This colour slow down an over-active heart; stimulate the spleen and the white blood cells, increasing immunity. Bring sleep. Soothe mental and emotional stress. Decrease sexual activity. Decrease sensitivity to pain and helps in detoxification.

Leonardo da Vinci proclaimed that you can increase the power of meditation ten-fold by meditating under the gentle rays of Violet, as found in Church windows.

Esoteric/magical: Elemental spirit. Divination and prophecy. Angels. Psychic abilities, divination, counter-acting negativity/black magic, reversing curses, psychic healing, psychic power, inspiration, meditation, spirituality, spiritual power, astral projection, third eye, compassion, counter-acting depression.

Preference for violet: Colours for meditation, contemplation, mysticism, spirituality and religion power.

A longing to ascend and dissolve polarities (purple consists of the active red and passive blue), to improve the world. Reservation, mystery and dignity. Soft, sensitive people with often paranormal abilities.

Aversion to violet: A person who has an aversion for violet / purple may have very serious attitude towards life; and may find it difficult to give dreams, fantasies, vague fears or memories a place in it.

May have tendency to rejection everything he regards as unnatural or unrealistic.

Purple and Scarlet

Purple is a combination of red and blue. The key property of purple that is used in colour therapy is the intense purification accorded by purple. Its main application is in detoxifying the body.

Scarlet and purple have opposite effects in colour therapy. For example, scarlet is a vasoconstrictor and raises the blood pressure while purple is a vasodilator and lowers the blood pressure.

Characteristics of Scarlet

- Scarlet stimulates kidney activity and the sexual mechanism.
- Scarlet helps in cases of impotency and frigidity when used in the genital area.
- Scarlet is useful in cases of scant menstruation.
- Scarlet is an arterial stimulant and a renal energizer.
- Scarlet is a genital exciter, an emmenagogue that promotes menstrual discharge, and a vasoconstrictor.
- It promotes libido in those with subnormal sex potency.

Characteristics of Purple
- Purple is used in excessive menstruation (opposite in effect to scarlet) If the bleeding is excessive, use indigo instead because it will reduce the bleeding more effectively.
- Purple has an analgesic, anti-pyretic, narcotic and hypnotic effect.
- Purple is indicated in malaria.
- Purple is the colour of anger, divinity and royalty.
- Purple is a venous stimulant.
- Purple gives authority, prestige, and distance;
- reduces heart pain, stiffness and cysts.

Diseases treated with Purple

Purple is considered by many to be a high vibrational colour. It is this high vibration which gives it its ability for purification. It is effective to use when strong detoxifying of the body is needed, as in the case of cancerous or pre-cancerous conditions. Purple is purifying to the body. It can be used to stimulate venous activity in the body. It can also be used for headaches.

The red-purple range is beneficial to balancing the polarities of the body. The blue- purple range is effective in helping to shrink (such as tumors) and to cool, easing inflammations. Because of its high vibration, purple should be used sparingly. Too much purple can create or aggravate depression. It can stagnate or suppress emotions - especially anger.

Healing properties: These are colours of transformation.

They heal melancholy, hysteria, delusions and alcohol addiction and bring spiritual insights and renewal. Decrease sensitivity to pain..

Esoteric/magical: Elemental spirit. Divination and prophecy. Angels. Psychic abilities, divination, counter-acting negativity/black magic, reversing curses, psychic healing, psychic power, inspiration, meditation, spirituality, spiritual power, compassion, counter-acting depression.

Preference for purple: Colours for meditation, contemplation, mysticism, spirituality and religion power. A longing to ascend and dissolve polarities (purple consists of the active red and passive blue), to improve the world. Reservation, mystery and dignity. Soft, sensitive people with often paranormal abilities.

Aversion to purple: A person who has an aversion for violet / purple may have very serious attitude towards life; and may find it difficult to give dreams, fantasies, vague fears or memories a place in it. May have tendency to rejection everything he regards as unnatural or unrealistic.

Magenta

Magenta is the colour of the highest order, connected with spirituality, meditation, and letting go. It is an agent for change, for the clearing out of old attitudes and obsessions, and for making a break with the post. Its complement is green.

Characteristics of Magenta

- Magenta energizes the adrenal glands, the heart action and the reproduction system.
- Magenta acts as a diuretic.
- Magenta is good for the treatment of the auric bodies.
- Magenta is a fine emotional stabilizer.

Healing properties: Strengthens contact with your life purpose. Stimulates adrenaline and heart activity.

Esoteric/magical: Scorpio-energy. Magnetism, to attract or speed up things, extra power, when immediate action and great spiritual power are needed, life purpose, life path.

Preference for magenta: Much energy and activity focused on achieving power and self-realization. Strong but controlled passions and emotions. Daring, ready to fight, willing to give everything for a goal. Can drive things too far and have fixed ideas.

Aversion to magenta: A person who has an aversion to magenta may feel overwhelmed by people with strong convictions or heavy emotions like jealousy; also may have difficulties with exposing deep emotions.

Lemon

The colour lemon is obtained by combining green and yellow. So, it has properties of both. It has important effects on the digestive system and the left hemisphere brain activity. The key application of the colour lemon in colour therapy is in mental stimulation.

Lemon is vitalizing and stimulating to the brain. Thus, it is effective in treating and alleviating conditions associated with it, such as Alzheimer's, senility, etc.

It can be used to help stimulate the brain's natural abilities. It always has a shade of green within the spectrum, and in lemon, the green works as a cleanser. Lemons assists us in bringing toxins to the surface so they can be cleaned out.

The toxins can be physical toxins as well as emotional toxins. Lemon is also effective in treating digestive problems and appendicitis. It facilitates the natural digestive process, helping the body assimilate nutrients more effectively. Lemon is good for tissues and bones.

Characteristics of Lemon Colour

- Lemon is a cerebral stimulant.
- Lemon stimulates the brain. It is also a sexual stimulant.
- Lemon activates the thymus gland and thus controls growth.
- Lemon being half green has the effect of a cleanser of the system, and being half yellow also has the effect of a motor stimulant to throw off morbid debris. Yellow and green are both cleansers and lemon has the quality of both.

Diseases Treated with Lemon
- Lemon strengthens the bone
- Bone growth
- Chronic conditions: Lemon has an antacid effect on the body, excellent for chronic conditions. It gives energy to the cells in the stage of resistance and exhaustion and helps overcome stress
- Cleanser of the system
- Coughing: use lemon as irradiative agent over the affected area
- Motor stimulant

Pink

Pink is soothing. It can be used for treating skin conditions and inflammations and the immune system.

Pink is a soothing colour on all levels, physical mental and emotional levels. It can be used to soothe conditions of anger and feelings of neglect. Pink can be used to awaken compassion, love, and purity. It can be used in meditation to discern greater truths. It is comforting to the emotional energies of the individual.

Physically, pink is most effective in the treatment of skin problems and conditions, especially when combined with aqua. It also stimulates the thymus gland and ease stresses upon the immune system of the body.

Healing properties: Heals grief and sadness. Restores youthfulness. Brings you in contact with your feelings.

Esoteric/magical: Softness and tenderness, romance, caring, nurturing, for children, youth, peace, friendship, femininity, emotional love, emotional healing.

Preference for pink: Regarded as a feminine colour. Pink symbolizes softness, sweetness, innocence, youthfulness and tenderness. Soft and kind people.

Aversion to pink: A person who has an aversion to pink may have a challenge with expressing soft, tender, female side.

Turquoise (Aqua)

No chakra is associated with turquoise. Turquoise combines the cleansing action of green and the soothing action of blue. It is soothing, purifying, and calming. Turquoise is used to combat inflammatory diseases and to boost the immune system. Its complement is red.

Characteristics of Turquoise

- Turquoise has the opposite effect of lemon; it is acid and tonic in its action.
- Turquoise is a prime skin-building colour and should be used after the pain from burns is relieved. Turquoise hastens the formation of new skin.
- Turquoise is a cerebral depressant for over-active mental patients.

Therapeutical Applications: Turquoise is important for respiratory system and in strengthening the metabolism. Aqua is cooling to the system. It can be beneficial in easing all feverish conditions and for balancing all systems of the body. It can also be used to cool and ease any inflammation. It combines both the beneficial effects of blue and green. It vitalizes all systems. It is also purifying. In treating febrile diseases, change to turquoise when the temperature is normal.

Aqua is useful in treating skin conditions, throat problems, and it is very effective for acute pain and earaches. It eases respiration problems. It is effective in treatment of asthma and bronchitis, especially with children. Regular colour breathing with aqua can prevent intense attacks of asthmatic conditions.

Healing properties: Increases intuition and sensitivity. Works disinfecting and antiseptic. Tones the general system. Builds the skin. Relaxes sensations of stress.

Esoteric/magical: Alterations, intellectual and intuitive insights, technique, inventions, originality, renewal, brotherhood, humanism.

Preference for turquoise: Just like the wide turquoise sea you don't want to feel restricted and you don't immediately bring to the surface what goes on in you; emotions can remain hidden. A colour for non-triviality, renewal, innovation and inventions, progressive technics, alternative ways of living together, humanity.

Aversion to turquoise: A person who has an aversion to turquoise may be looking for solidity and security in society, especially in marriage. Also, may be reluctant to think originally or to walk new paths.

Ultraviolet

Characteristics of Ultraviolet
Physical:
- Ultra-violet has a chemical and bacteriocidal action on the blood and tissues of the body. It breaks down the bacterial toxins and helps the white blood cells in their phagocytic action.
- Ultra-violet's chemical reaction depends upon its vitamin reaction in the system. Vitamins A, B, C, D and E are affected by the ultra-violet light.
- Ultra-violet plays a great part in the calcium phosphorus balance and in iron and iodine fixation.
- Ultra-violet accelerates the lymphatic and circulatory activities.
- Ultra-violet normalizes all metabolism and glandular activities.
- Ultra-violet stimulates antibody production and immunizes the body against disease.
- Ultra-violet has a stimulating action on the Sympathetic System. It, however, acts as a sedative to pain.
- Ultra-violet is good for the heart and the lungs.

Diseases Treated with Ultra-Violet
- Goiter
- Gonorrhea
- Heart
- Lungs
- Rickets
- Syphilis
- Ulcer
- Wounds

Brown

Brown is an earthy colour. It grounds, stabilizes and neutralizes. It is an effective colour in healing.

Brown is especially effective in stabilizing overexcited states. It calms and grounds emotions and extreme mental conditions. Brown can help awaken common sense and discrimination. It brings us back down to earth.

Brown is effective for any kind of spaceness. When it shows up in the human aura, brown may indicate a need for grounding. When the aura takes the shade of brown, it will often reflect infection in the body or that area of the body in which it overlays in the aura.

Brown can be used to stabilize all systems. It is useful in cases of hyperactivity with children, especially with combinations of colours in the rust to deep brown range.

Too much exposure to brown may make one's personality coarser.

Esoteric/magical: Elemental earth. The planet-spirit Saturn. Stability, grounding, conservation, protection of household, family and pets, healing animals, finding lost objects, material constructions, material increase, to make relationships solid, to increase decisiveness and concentration, attracting help in financial crisis.

Preference for brown: An earthly colour for practical people with a preference for natural, tribal and primitive things, solidity and simplicity.

Brown can be warm and cosy but also depressing. Family-life persons, stable people, loyal friends.

Aversion to brown: A person who has an aversion to brown may feel an aversion against normal, boring, trivial life; may not feel connected with his roots (home-land, family, etc); may experience instability in health and attitude.

Grey

Esoteric/magical: Neutralizing negative influences, erasing or cancelling situations, causing stalemates

Preference for grey: Very neutral and indifferent, non-expressive. It can be deliberate, but also lifeless, fixed, depressed and apathic. Reserved, cool people; unwilling to expose themselves or to have obligations. Grey can be refined and tactful.

Aversion to grey: A person who has an aversion to grey may prefers to be straight to the point, no time for political and tactical attitudes. Demands clarity, a knowing where one stands.

Gold

Gold is an important colour in oriental healing. Its principal property is in strengthening and amplifying. Gold is very useful in increasing the self-consciousness. It has beneficial effect on the immune system and on the cardiac conditions.

Gold is a colour that can strengthen the energies associated with the entire immune system. It can be used with other colours to amplify the effects without overexciting the system. It is very strengthening to the heart. It is effective to use in regard to all cardiac problems, especially as a powerful tonic after heart surgery.

Gold is a powerful stimulant to the immune system of the body.

It helps awaken the individual's own healing abilities to assist the body in restoring homeostasis. It can also awaken renewed enthusiasm.

Gold is also believed to improve libido, especially in women. Gold also harmonizes the mind and affect the endocrine systems. In ayurveda, gold is believed to affect the ojas.

Ojas is the by-product of a healthy, efficient, contented physiology. It is the "juice" that remains after food has been properly digested and assimilated. When you are producing ojas, it means all your organs have integrated vitality and you are receiving the nourishment your mind and body need. Your whole being hums with good vibrations because you are producing and feeling bliss, not pain. However, when your agni isn't working properly, you don't produce ojas. Instead food, thoughts, and feelings turn into ama.

Ojas is the subtle glue that cements the body, mind and spirit together, integrating them into a functioning individual.

Esoteric/magical: Absolute authority, (self)confidence, creativity, perfection, solar energies, male energy, financial riches, investments, luxury, winning, worldly power, magical power, overcoming bad habits/addictions

Black

Black is a protective colour. It is grounding and calming, especially to extremely sensitive individuals. It activates the magnetic or feminine energies of the body, strengthening them.

Black is the spiritual colour for some religions; but it is the colour of death for others. It promotes resistance, obstruction, opposition, and enmity. It wards off hatred and negative emotions. Black is most effective when used in conjunction with white, balancing the polarities of the individual, especially in cases where the individual seems to be losing control.

It can activate the subconscious mind which can put life and all of its craziness into proper perspective. It should rarely be used by itself, but always in combination with another colour.

Black should be used sparingly, as too much black can cause depression or aggravate such emotional/mental conditions. Black also increases fear, suspicion and paranoia.

Esoteric/magical: Elemental earth. Deities of the underworld. Repel/banish evil and negativity, protection, banishing, binding, breaking free from bad habits/addictions, deep meditation, opens up deep unconscious levels.

Preference for black: Symbolizes seriousness, darkness, depression, death, mourning, mystery, secrecy, occultism, a standing apart from or revolting against triviality, provocation, underground, underworld, things that have to remain hidden, nothingness as the great source of all creation, the need to keep your energy with you. Black is a colour for extremes, everything and nothing. People who foremost trust themselves.

Aversion to black: A person who has an aversion to black may have fear for the unknown, or fear for the abuse of power. Desires to become free from all kinds of dependency, blockages, hindrances; to throw off shackles.

White

White, or full colour spectrum white colour, contains the entire light spectrum. Thus it influences all systems of the body. This is the basis for light therapy.

White is strengthening. It is cleansing and purifying to the entire energy system. It promotes purity, virtue and spirituality. White is nurturing; heals fevers, infections and pain; calms the heart, mind, nerves and emotions; and promotes vitality and supportive feelings.

White can awaken greater creativity. When in doubt as to what colour to use, you can seldom go wrong with white.

It is beneficial to begin and end a colour therapy session with white to stabilize the energy system of the individual and to give it an overall boost. It amplifies the effects of any other colour used with it in a healing session.

If used in excess, white light causes passivity, lethargy, hypersensitivity, and inhibitions.

Healing properties: White is the perfect colour; for it is all colours, in perfect balance and harmony. It is the colour of the awakened Spirit; the light of perfection; the light of the Cosmic Consciousness , the Divine Light.

Just about everyone has heard of surrounding people with the "White Light of Healing and Protection." White light raises the vibration of one's consciousness and the body, bringing harmony in all aspects of one's life. Directing white into to a part of the body that needs healing is one of the fastest ways to bring about healing.

Esoteric/magical: Purification and cleaning on all levels, contact with higher self and spiritual helpers, (inner) peace, aura-healing, truth seeking, consecration, spiritual enlightenment, protection against negativity by raising your vibration, breaking curses, exorcism, meditation, divination, inspiration, clairvoyance, invoking spirits White can be a replacement for any other colour your magic requires.

Preference for white: White points at innocence, purity, virginity, cleanliness, freshness, simplicity, nothingness, oneness and completion, truth. In certain cultures white is the colour of death and mourning.

Aversion to white: A person who has an aversion to white colour is foremost or solely interested in 'realistic' and tangible things, not in illusions or things that are beyond seeing or understanding. Knows and accepts the own imperfection and does not wish to achieve perfection

Colour Pages

Now that we have a basic understanding of colours will be easy improve our daily mood or improve the way we feel now by simply watching and focusing on a colour. Another way is to close the eyes and imagine the colour for five to ten minutes. I added a page for each colour so will be easier to watch, focus, think or meditate.

Before you begin your mediation, mentally assess your thoughts and your physical feelings. Do you have a relationship issue that is troubling you? Focus on red and your root chakra. Are you having trouble speaking up for yourself? Focus on the colour blue and your throat chakra. If you are feeling a physical weakness anywhere in your body, focus on the colour and chakra that affects those conditions.

Try an overall colour meditation. Sit or lie down in a comfortable position in a quiet room. Take a few deep cleansing breaths. Start breathing slowly and evenly. Visualize a golden light over your head and draw the light down through your body, all the way to your toes. Allow the light to illuminate every aspect of your being. When you feel completely relaxed, begin meditating on each chakra and its colour. Start at your root chakra, which is red, and focus on the aspects of that chakra while you visualize the colour red. Continue focusing on each colour and chakra until you reach the crown chakra. Finish your meditation by taking a few more deep cleansing breaths. Once again, visualize your being with golden light before you come out of your meditative state.

Colours, like features, follow the changes of the emotions. -
Pablo Picasso

Colour	Chakra	Chakra location	Alleged function
Red	First	Base of the spine	Grounding and Survival
Orange	Second	Lower abdomen, genitals	Emotions, sexuality
Yellow	Third	Solar plexus	Power, ego
Green	Fourth	Heart	Love, sense of responsibility
Blue	Fifth	Throat	Physical and spiritual communication
Indigo	Sixth	Just above the center of the brow, middle of forehead	Forgiveness, compassion, understanding
Violet	Seventh	Crown of the head	Connection with universal energies, transmission of ideas and information

Please be aware that no complementary therapy should be considered as an alternative to professional medical advice where necessary and no properly qualified complementary therapist would suggest that, neither would they suggest that you stop taking your medication etc. If you are taking medication you should consult the prescribing professional before you stop taking it.

Resources:

1. Klotsche C. Colour Medicine. Arizona: Light Technology Publishing; 1993.
2. Azeemi, Khawaja Shamsuddin. Colour Therapy. Karachi: Al-Kitab Publications; 1999.
3. Hassan M. Chromopathy. Peshawar: Institute of Chromopathy; 2000.
4. Azeemi, S. T.; Raza, S. M. (2005). "A Critical Analysis of Chromotherapy and Its Scientific Evolution
5. Pleasanton A. Blue and Sun Light. Philadelphia: Claxton, Reuser & Haffelfinger; 1876.
6. Babbitt E. Principles of Light and Colour. MT, USA: Kessinger Publishing; 1942
7. Qalander B. 1979. LOH-O-QALAM, Maktaba Tajuddin Baba Auliya, Karachi.
8. Schauss AG. Tranquilizing effect of colour reduces aggressive behaviour and potential violence. J Orthomol Psych. 1979;4:218–21.
9. Walker M. Power of Colours. NY, USA: Avery Publishing Group; 1990.
10. Angie Arkin, Intuitive Healer, www.beyourownhealer.com
11. Jasmine Sky, The Dreaming Goddess, www.thedreaminggoddess.com

P.V. Mihalache

ABOUT THE AUTHOR

Paul Valentin Mihalache is a Romanian writer, born 04/06/1986, who lives in London, United Kingdom, since 2010. With a Bachelor Degree in Physical Education and Sports and a PhD in Sports Activities he dedicated his life and career to sport, especially to football.

He is a Level 4 FA Football Referee since 2014 , officiating in the United Counties Football League, Barclays U18 Premier League, Women's Super League and others Midlands and Bedfordshire Leagues.

With great experience as PE teacher, personal trainer and fitness instructor he started in 2015 to write "The Art of Happiness" series. The books are aiming to deliver information on how to achieve a healthy lifestyle

Chromotherapy – Colours and Well-being -" is the 2rd of the series, following "Happiness Guide – How to boost your Serotonin level-"

www.ingramcontent.com/pod-product-compliance
Lightning Source LLC
Chambersburg PA
CBHW061158180526
45170CB00002B/850